The Proven Acne Natural Remedies And Natural Cures Exposed

Plethora of Natural Healing Secretes For
Acne and pimples You can Use without Any
Drug or surgery; and Without Side Effects

Dr. Art T Dash, M.Sc., M.S., Ph.D.,

Copy Right: 2012

Yesterday is but a dream, tomorrow is but a vision.
But today well-lived
makes every yesterday a dream of happiness and
every tomorrow a vision
of hope. Look well, therefore, to this day

A

Sanskrit Proverb

DISCLAIMER

This book is not intended to diagnose, treat, or replace the service of a doctor or a healthcare personal. If you have any health conditions or are under a doctor's care, you must consult your physician or a health care professional before you apply any of the recommendations set forth in the pages of this book.

All information available in this book is for educational purposes only and none of the stated products have been FDA approved. Any application of the recommendations mentioned in this book is at the reader's discretion and sole risk.

The publication is offered "as is" without warranty of any kind either expressed or implied, including but not limited to, the implied warranties of merchantability, suitability for a particular purpose or non-infringement. Descriptions of or reference to products or publications does not imply endorsement of that product or publication.

ITNTRODUCTION

For those who have bad acne, find a while to unwind and make certain you receive enough sleep. Acne could be triggered by stress and exhaustion. You most likely have little treatments for what really causes you stress, but you will find a method to balance your existence to ensure that it's not your primary preoccupation.

Purchasing an oil-free, skin doctor-approved moisturizer in it is important for reducing acne. Using the right oil-free moisturizer in it you can have smooth skin with no side-effect of more acne. If you don't make use of an oil-free moisturizer in it, there's a significantly greater chance your pores can get clogged and, thus, result in a breakout of acne.

To avoid acne, a great hygiene is essential. Washing the face carefully might help; however, you also need to give consideration as to what touches the face. For example, would you clean your pillow situation or sheets regularly? You need to clean these once per week to make certain they don't retain any oil out of your skin.

The easiest method to prevent acne breakouts and also hardwearing is to keep your hands off the face. Many people touch their face many occasions each day, and hands are filled with bacteria that will get into pores around the face. Avoid touching the face area with hands to help keep dirt, oil and bacteria from inflaming facial pores.

For those who have a far more severe type of acne, use an aspirin mask each time you receive a pimple in your face. Aspirin has numerous soothing qualities, which could lessen the time acne remain on the face and expedite the recovery process. It will help you overcome your acne using the level of comfort that you want.

To prevent the likelihood of making more acne trouble for yourself, feel, as this the face. Touching the face transfers grime and bacteria for your pores, and may also cause already inflamed areas being much more inflamed. Also avoid popping any acne or blemishes together with your bare fingers, because they are only going to complicate matters.

Although energy drinks are very efficient to provide you with the extra kick that you need for your work day, they can contribute to acne. These drinks are filled with a plethora of sugar and caffeine, which can expedite the formation of acne and cause new pimples to form. Avoid your energy drink intake to improve your skin. If you have bad acne, find some time to relax and make sure you get enough sleep. Acne can be caused by stress and exhaustion. You probably have very little control over what actually causes you stress, but you can find a way to balance your life so that it is not your main preoccupation.
.

To avoid the chance of creating more acne, a great hygiene is essential. Washing the face carefully might help; however, you also need to give consideration as to what touches the face. For example, would you clean your pillow situation or sheets so that they don't retain any oil out of your skin regularly? You need to clean these once per week regularly to prevent acne further progressing.

Table of Contents

What is Acne?

Acne is an inflammatory condition of the skin where sebaceous glands (oil glands) in the skin excrete excessive amount of sebum causing pores to become plugged, usually resulting in outbreak of lesions commonly called whiteheads, blackheads, and pustules. Acne lesions normally occur where sebaceous glands are most numerous and active, such as the face, neck, chest, chin, shoulders, back. Although acne is not a life threatening health problem, it can be a source of considerable emotional distress. Severe acne can cause permanent scarring.

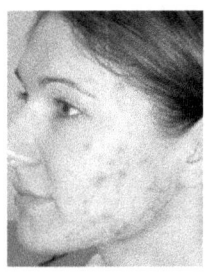

How Does Acne Develop?

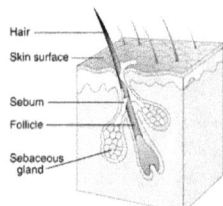

Acne is an inflammatory condition of the skin where sebaceous glands in the skin excrete excessive amount of sebum causing pores to become plugged resulting in whiteheads, blackheads, and inflamed pustules.

Sebum that is produced by sebaceous glands is necessary to protect the skin from elements and to keep it moist. Under certain conditions sebaceous glands produce excessive sebum and excrete increased production of keratin (a protective protein that covers the skin.) Hair, excessive sebum and keratin along with bacteria and other substances fill the narrow follicles causing a plug signaling an early onslaught of acne. Besides others, some of the primary conditions causing acne are hormonal changes during adolescence, and fluctuating hormones.

Hormones play a significant role in causing acne. It is the androgenic (male) sex hormones, for instance testosterone, which produce an increase in sebaceous gland outputs clogging their pores and allowing the bacterial infection occur, an onset of the acne. These hormonal changes and fluctuations occur during adolescents both male and female, and during pregnancy, that cause excessive production of sebum that clog pores, encouraging bacteria to develop resulting in formation of acne. Typically, the hormone levels rise during adolescence. While acne is more prevalent in in adolescents (more than 80 % of those between the ages of 12 and 21 are inflicted), it now appears in increasing frequencies in adults. The study shows that the tendency to develop acne can be genetically inherited from parents.

The cause of acne in newborns is not clearly understood, but researchers theorize that it may be due to the transfer through the placenta of hormones from the mother or of acne-causing medications (i.e., lithium, and phenytoin) that the mother may have been using. Sex hormones and fluctuating hormones are not the only causative factors for acne, there are other causative factors, such as poor nutrition, bad fats, improper foods, sugar, and processed foods. All these not only accelerate the skin inflammation and acne, but also aggravate the condition.

Symptoms

The symptoms of acne are characterized by each of the following conditions that appear in face, cheek, chin, chest, or back.

• Papules: inflamed lesions that appear as small, pink bums on the skin

• Pustules (pimples): inflamed pus filled painful lesions, red at the base

• Cysts and nodules: large inflamed pus-filled lesions, causing pain and scarring

• Blackheads, whiteheads, and/or oily skin

DIAGRAM OF A TYPICAL PIMPLE

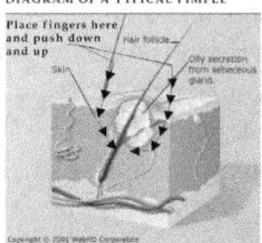

Primary Causes

• **Genetics**

• **Puberty**: during this time there is an excessive production of androgenic (male) sex hormones that increase sebaceous gland activity leading to clogged pores.

• **Diets** (poor diets): avoid or substantially reduce diets consisting of saturated fats (e.g., milk, diary products, meat, fried foods, pastry, hydrogenated fats, excess sugar, which potentiates the effect of fats, refined carbohydrates, chocolate, caffeine (cola, tea, coffee)), pops, alcohol, processed foods (contain trans fats), lack of vegetables. If you want to stay healthy, passionately avoid these diets.

• **Nutritional Deficiencies**: zinc, B6 (birth control medications depletes B6), malabsorption (lack of hydrochloric acid reduces zinc absorption), or antioxidants depletion due to medications and drugs,

• **Food** sensitivities or allergies

• **Hormonal** fluctuations or imbalance

- **Poor elimination**: Bowel lesion (thinning) due to bad diets or stress caused by constipation, liver congestion or toxicity; overstressed kidney function
- **Steroids**, oral contraceptives, cosmetics, lack of exercise
- **Candida and/or yeast overgrowth**

Diagnosis:

In order to determine proper therapy for acne one should perform the following tests:
- Food allergies and/or food sensitivities
- Nutritional Deficiency Testing: blood/urine/hair analysis
- Stool/blood analysis for yeast overgrowth
- Blood sugar test
- Saliva hormone analysis for estrogen/progesterone/testosterone balance

Treatment

Diet

Drink a glass of clean water every two waking hours to flush toxin out of the system and to maintain good health. This is very essential for tissue cleansing and elimination. In some cases it is essential to avoid foods rich in iodine, such as shellfish, seafood, and iodized table salt, because iodine may worsen acne.

It is ideal for acne suffers to consume basic and unprocessed foods. The ideal diet must include dark green, and yellow orange colored fruits and vegetables, are particularly beneficial, since they contain beta carotene which helps maintain and restore the skin take them raw or lightly cooked or steamed to preserve their beneficial nutrients and fiber. Plenty of fresh non-citrus fruits, and fresh vegetable juice, and seafood soups are very beneficial.

Consume enough fibrous foods, such as salba, prune juice. A two tablespoons of grounded salba twice daily not only provides adequate amount of fiber for proper elimination, but it also contains omega-3 fatty acids which has numerous health benefits, including cancer, heart disease, stroke, arthritis,. Take also nuts, and seeds, such as almonds, sunflower seeds, walnuts, and pumpkin seeds for their zinc.

You don't necessarily need meat for protein. There are excellent protein sources, such as beans, peas, lentil, eggs; and seaweeds are beneficial for their high iodine content. If you want animal protein take cold water fish like cod, salmon, mackerel, herring, and sardines which are extremely beneficial for health since these protein sources are rich in omega-3 fatty acids essential for the maintenance of good health.

If you must eat meat protein, then you must find meat products free of hormone and antibiotics, like grass-fed beef, free range chicken.

Foods To Avoid

Eliminate junk and processed foods, such as luncheon meat, bacon, sausage, hotdogs, fried foods, chips, pops, energy drinks, and candies, because these foods are large sources of toxins; and loaded with sugar, salt, dangerous preservatives and chemicals that are extremely harmful for health. Avoid sugar and sugary products, since they encourage oil production which is conducive to bacteria and yeast.

Check for the food allergies. Adult acne is generally an allergic reaction or sensitivity to certain foods. Although any food can cause an allergic reaction, by far the most common triggers are diary and dairy products, wheat, sugars or sugary products, chocolate, and corn, breakfast cereals.

An internal acidic environment is conducive to acne, thus avoid alcohol, sugar, chocolate, fried foods, candies, pops, and meat products.

Eliminate saturated fats (i.e., milk, and all dairy products), trans fats (processed foods, fried foods, fast foods, margarine), refined carbohydrates (sugar, white bread, pops, breakfast cereals), hydrogenated fats (i.e., margarine, vegetable shortening, generally made by hydrogenating unsaturated fats and making them partially saturated). These hydrogenated fats are entirely unnatural to the body and should be avoided altogether, if possible. Commercial baked goods often contain up to 20 % fat should be strictly avoided. Avoid Canola oil and vegetable oils. Use extra virgin olive oil and extra virgin coconut oil.

Detoxification

Detoxification help cleanses the body of toxins, and poisons accumulated over the years due to the consumption of bad foods, such as processed foods, sugar, pops, fried foods, tran fats, saturated fats, hydrogenated fats, etc. Detoxifying your entire system (i.e., blood, liver, kidneys, and bladder) a couple of times a year would help to maintain good health and protect you from degenerative diseases, as well. There are various ingredients available in Health Food stores for detoxifying your body, also internet websites. However, I strongly advise you to discuss with a healthcare professional before you decide to detoxify your system. Furthermore, you may find that your situations, (including acne), worsen immediately after following the detoxification therapies, because your body, (or skin), eliminating toxins at a faster rate than usual. Once the toxins are eliminated, your bodily conditions, including acne, should be reduced or eliminated. If you do not wish to try these ingredients, you may adopt the following procedures. Again if you have conditions, you are strongly advised to consult a healthcare professional.

Fasting is one of the best known procedures to detoxifying the system. There are various kinds of fasting:
- **Water fast**
- **Juice fast**

• **Mono fast**

Water fast is the best form of detoxification that will sweep away the toxic build-up. Drink only pure water for three days. It is better to do the fasting under the supervision of a healthcare professional.

Juice fast may be more welcomed, since some may find water fast more tiring. Don't juice fast on store bought juices. They are processed and may contain harmful chemicals or more sodium. Fast on fresh juice made from: carrots, apples, and beets with their tops, papaya, as well as green drinks, including spirulina, wheatgrass, barley grass, chlorella). This will cleanse the system.

Mono fast: eat only one kind of food (or a particular juice) whole week. may be one kind of fruit, or vegetable, or just rice, or just beans....etc.

For more information see the section on Detoxification. Detoxification will help cleanse the body and is especially supportive of an acne cleanse. See alternative natural remedies: http://www.alternativenaturalremedies.com

Conventional Therapies

Your doctor may prescribe topical, and/or oral medications:

Topical: Topical medications are those applied directly to skin. They are available in many forms, including gels, lotions, cream, or pads. The most commonly used topical medications are:

Benzoyl peroxide, glycolic acid, synthetic vitamin A derivatives, and Antibiotics.

Oral: Antibiotics (work by killing bacteria and reducing inflammation), Isotretinoin (works by reducing the size of oil glands and lowering sebum production).

Side Effects: People using isotretinoin experience serious side effects, such as

• Suicidal tendencies,
• Dry eyes, mouth, lips, nose, or skin
• Itching

- Nosebleeds
- Muscle aches
- Sensitive to sun
- Poor night vision
- Change in liver function
- Increase in cholesterol and triglyceride levels
- Antibiotics also cause several serious side effects, including destruction of intestinal flora and vaginal flora which makes the patients
vulnerable to infectious diseases

Acidophilus & Bifidus or Probiotics

As it is mentioned above, antibiotics destroy beneficial bacteria in intestines and vaginal flora. In order to protect these beneficial bacteria, patients taking antibiotics should be advised to take Acidophilus & Bifidus or probiotics.

L-carnitine

Researchers in Greece have shown that a large group of people who had side effects from using isotretinoin got better by taking L-carnitine compared to those who took a placebo.

Surgery and other procedures are used, such as steroid injection of large acne, depending on the severity of cases.

Consult with your doctor. But our interest here is based on

Natural Remedies

Niacinamide face cleansing pads are effective and simple way to keep acne away. Just place a pad on the pimple and watch it fade away. Lavender Oil helps prevent skin drying. Niacinamide pads are also known as Nicotinamide pads or Vit   B3   pads.

Give them a try and you will be pleasantly surprised.

Natural Supplements for Acne Cure

Many dietary deficiencies contribute to inflammation, and inflammation is a major factor of acne.

Take high potency multiple vitamin rich in trace minerals (calcium, magnesium, potassium ;...). Take Vitamin A (30,000 – 50,000 IU) twice daily. Vitamin C (500 – 1000 mg 3 times daily): antioxidant, stress reducer, Chromium (400 mcg) daily with meals. It regulates blood sugar. High blood sugar peaks may contribute to acne. They all provide antioxidant protection against free radical damage; and help cleanse the body from toxicity, and is especially supportive of acne cleanse. Here are some important nutrients that will help nourish the body to fight diseases, including acne.

Omega-3 fatty acids:

Reduce inflammation throughout your body by reducing the production of cytokines, messenger chemicals involved in the inflammatory response. Walnuts, salmon and salba are excellent dietary sources. You can also purchase a good Omega-3 supplement, Fish Oil supplement, or take a tablespoon of cod liver oil each day. Sounds gross, but there are lemon-flavored cod liver oils on the market that really aren't unpleasant, and can help make your skin glow! You can find them sold in capsule form in any health food store.

Calcium, Magnesium and Vitamin D:

Calcium: Among many other health reasons for taking calcium, calcium helps to soothe nerves.

Magnesium aids in the absorption of calcium, and also has many other important health benefits, such as high blood pressure and heart health.

Vitamin D aids in the absorption of calcium, as well, and Vitamin D deficiencies can be a source of systemic inflammation in many people. Vitamin D is a panacea. It prevents every disease you can name, such as heart disease, cancer, stroke, diabetes, cognitive dementia; develop strong bones, Alz's and Parkinson's disease, etc

Vitamin A:

Vitamin A aids in the skin-healing process, and it is contained in your fish oil supplement. However, you can take 25,000 units twice a day to aid in healing.

Vitamin B6: is effective in premenstrual acne. Take a 50 mg B-complex before and during premenstrual flare-ups.

Vitamin E-Complex: consisting of tocopherols and tocotrienols, enhances the beneficial effects of selenium and vitamin A. Dose: 400 IU or 800 IU. Start first with 400 IU, then slowly increase to 800 IU

Selenium, a trace mineral, is useful in reducing the inflammation of acne. Dose: 200 mcg, daily. Check whether your multivitamin contains 200 mcg of selenium.

Zinc:

This little miracle aids in the healing process and helps prevent scarring. How's that for a simple home treatment for acne?

Take 50 mg with 5 mg copper, because zinc can cause a slight deficiency in copper.

Hydrate!

There are lots of formulas for how much water a certain person with a certain body weight under certain conditions needs. A simple rule is to drink 8 glasses of 8 ounce glass of water a day that you've always known you're supposed to drink. Just do it! Coffee, tea, soft drinks, energy drinks, juices won't do; just water.

-**Probiotics** to replenish the beneficial bacteria in intestine and/or vagina.

Without adequate nutrition, the body will rebel to produce excessive sebum, clogging pores, and reducing the ability for your skin to heal and fight bacteria.

Primary Therapeutic Recommendations

Here are some of the potent ingredients which can greatly help reduce acne formation. First start with the first one then see what the effect is. If the condition improves within a month or six weeks, continue with it until it is eliminated; otherwise add to it the next ingredient, and so on.

- **chasteberry** (vitex).....................180 mg, a standardize vitex extract (0.6 % aucubin or 0.5 % agnuside) or 40 drops daily of vitex tincture use this at least for six weeks. If there is noticeable improvement, continue with it as long as it remains beneficial; otherwise add to it the next ingredient.

Vitex (Agnus-Castus) is an excellent hormone balancer which can help reduce acne formation in both men and women. Recent several clinical studies reported that vitex is a potent herbal treatment for infertility, female hormonal imbalance, ovulatory irregularity, anovulation, amenorrhea, menstrual disorders, and other disorders related to hormone function in women.

Vitex is effective in stimulating and normalizing hypothalamus and pituitary gland functions. It also helps regulate and balance female hormone production. It is also called Monk's Pepper, may be because, it reduces libido in men and women. In ancient times, its flowers were sprinkled on Queens's bed so that she can keep her chastity.

- **Zinc (mentioned earlier)**: for the treatment of acne, take 40 to 50 mg twice daily with meals for two or three months, then reduce the dosage to 25 mg twice daily for long-term supplementation. You must take zinc with 3 to 5 mg of copper. Don't use zinc sulfate, since it is not readily absorbed.

Zinc is one of the most important minerals to use for the treatment of acne. It is effective in reducing build up of DHT and promotes skin healing. It may take up to three months before you notice any benefits. Do not use zinc sulfate. It is not readily absorbed.

Here are some other health benefits of zinc—supports a healthy immune system—

helps wound healing—heals skin ulcers, bed sores, skin lesions—helps maintain

sense of taste and smell—needed in DNA (the cells genetic material)—essential for

cell division—supports growth and development during pregnancy and adolescence-

helps support normal semen production and maintain testosterone levels.

Vegetarians should use zinc supplement

- **EFA** (essential fatty acids) has numerous health benefits, including heart health, arthritis, strokes. Essential fatty acid formulations, such as Omega 3-6-9 contain all the essential mixture of flax oil, fish oil, and other relevant ingredients are beneficial for the treatment of acne and reduce skin inflammation..

Dosage: follow the direction as indicated in the container or as suggested by a health-care professional.

- **Neem** (Azadirachta indica) tree is indigenous to India. Traditionally its leafs and bark have been used in Ayurvedic medicines for myriads of diseases. Decades of research led to believe that it is a panacea for all chronic degenerative diseases. Numerous scientific studies have documented the Neem's immune enhancement properties as a booster of the macrophage's effectiveness. Various scientific studies have shown that Neem boosts the immune system be energizing lymphocytes cells to react to infection and other challenges to body's immunity.

External applications of neem oil in skin diseases are highly effective, because of its antiseptic properties. Preparations from the leaves oil of the tree are used as antiseptics The antibacterial properties of Neem make it highly effective to fight most epidermal dysfunctions, such as acne, psoriasis, eczema.

Dosage: two capsules three times daily with meals or as advised by a health-care Provider. Also put neem oil right onto the acne spots before bed.

- **Haemafine** Syrup is an herbal remedy for all types of skin diseases through blood purification. It not only gives a natural glow to the skin, but also improves complexion and gives an ultimate cure for acne, pimple, eczema, psoriasis, and other skin conditions, including nose bleeding.

Dosage: two teaspoons 2-3 times daily or as directed by a healthcare practitioner.

Note: not suitable for diabetic patients.

- **Ayurvedic Neem Balm**: The potent power of Neem oil combined with several other active ingredients forms the Ayurvedic Neem Balm, which has been traditionally used by Ayurvedic specialists to treat a wide variety of problem skin conditions, such as acne, psoriasis, eczema, septic sores, burns, insect bites, athletic foot, rashes, bruises, fungal infections, haemorrhoids, hives, inflammation, joint pain, muscle sores, warts and skin ulcers. It tones and promotes dry, itchy, wrinkled skin making it soft, moist and youthful. It nourishes, strengthens, and protects nails. You can also find Neem capsules to take them orally.

- **Amla:** is Indian gooseberry which has been used in Ayurvedic medicines over 5,000 years. It is a remedy for numerous diseases, such as fortifies liver, purifies blood, help skin diseases, used in hair care, reduce cholesterol, enhances fertility, regulates blood sugar, helps diabetes, improves eye sight, prevents cataract and macular degeneration, diarrhea and dysentery, rid the body of toxins etc.

- **Most importantly,** if you take Amla in combination with Neem, it can help clear out pimples that are caused due to impure blood. As mentioned above, Amla purifies and cleans the blood..

There are several types of green food supplements are available in health food stores, such as spirulina, sun chlorella, barley grass, or a combination of all of these and other green super foods that are extremely helpful for health.

- **Tea Tree Oil**: Tea tree oil comes from melaleuca tree is native to Australia. Tea Tree Oil is effective in the treatment of ailments described below.

Skin Care: acne, abscess, athlete's foot, blisters, burns, cold sores, dandruff, herpes, insect bites, oily skin, rashes, spots, warts and wounds. Tea Tree Oil also helps in the areas of health:

Genito-urinary system: thrush, vaginitis, cystitis,

It also helps allay the conditions, such as colds, flu, infectious illness like chicken pox,

It is also anti-fungal and anti-viral.

Use: apply it by dabbing it onto blemishes twice daily. It is quite potent; test it on small area teabenzyl peroxide, but without the drying side effects.

- **Acnenil**--is a safe Ayurvedic herbal skin care product which is used to eliminate

acne, improve skin texture, and add a healthy glow to the complexion.

Burdock Root (Arctinum lappa):

Dose: Take 300 to 500 mg of the capsule form, 30 drops of tincture or 1 cup of tea 3 times daily. It works as a blood purifier and a detoxifier, and it improves elimination. It also has hormone-balancing properties. Take it for a minimum of 8 weeks.

Green Tea – has antibacterial properties and antioxidants. It is also becoming very popular as an aid to reducing weight. The catechins in green tea help to regulate your hormonal levels, specifically the epigallocatechin gallate (EGGG). Green Tea when used for treating acne can be iaBenzoyl peroxide which is a popular medication for acne. As a drink the antioxidants in green tea help in detoxification and reducing inflammation.

Home Remedies

Indian Acne Home Cure: using water, make a paste with a teaspoon of turmeric powder and a teaspoon of sandalwood powder. Put it on your acne and it will clear up. This is commonly used for acne treatment in India. You can find sandalwood powder online or an Indian grocery store.

Lemon and Orange peel – contain citric acid which has an anti-bacterial effect by inhibiting the growth of the bacteria which would otherwise be exacerbating the acne. The orange peel can be applied to the acne area either by rubbing as a peel or by crushing with water and mixing with gram flour is an effective face scrub which will help to cleanse the skin of excess sebum.

Homeopathy

Generally a professional homeopath may recommend a remedy or remedies by taking into account of several factors, such as patient's constitutional type, his or her physical, emotional, and intellectual make up, including, of course, the symptoms of the disease. A clinically experienced homeopath assesses all these factors to determine the appropriate remedy or a combination of homeopathic remedies that matches all aspects of the particular patient.

As regards as acne is concerned, he may recommend one or more of the following remedies that is appropriate to a particular patient. Normally a potency of 6x, 12x, 6C or 30C is used. These remedies come in sugar pills or liquids. Keep three or five pellets or one pump under the tongue, if it is liquid. If the recommended remedy improves your condition, discontinue using it, otherwise add other remedies from the following.

Belladonna—-has marked action on the vascular system, skin, and glands and is always associated with hot red skin, flushed face and glaring eyes; in particular it is used for inflamed pustular acne with red lesions deep in the skin and no pus showing that improves with cold applications.

Calcarea Sulphurica— is effective for the treatment of eczema, torpid glandular
swelling, cystic tumors, Fibroids; and cystic acne or chronic acne with yellow
discharge and skin affections with yellow scabs.

Calendula—is used for skin conditions involving pustules or blisters.

Hepar Sulphur (*Hepar Sulphuris Calcareum*)—unhealthy skin, chapped skin with deep cracks on hands and feet, papules prone to suppurate, acne in youth, several pus-filled spots that are painful if touched, and skin lesions feel better with a warm compress.

Kali Bichromicum—-is a remedy for acne, popular eruptions, pustular eruptions resembling smallpox with burning and itching pains.

Kali Bromatum — for deep acne, especially on face and forehead, in persons who are chilled and nervous, pustules, itching is worst on chest, shoulders, and face.

Pulsatila — -is a remedy for acne associated with the hormonal changes during puberty, menstrual cycle or menopause. ,

Sulphur — usual homeopathic remedy for acne on nose, dandruff of scalp and eyebrows, including reddish, inflamed acne pustules that may be itchy or very sore, eruptions worse with washing and heat.

Often this remedy is alternated with the specific indicated remedy. For instance, use the indicated remedy for two or three weeks, then sulphur one week. Repeat this process until the condition clears.

You may look at other homeopathic remedies for acne, such as **Silica** (for white pustules), **Thuja, Antimon, Hydrocot, Cimicif, Berb. Aquif**.

Other Therapeutic Agents

Saw palmetto (*serenoa repens*) inhibits DHT of the sebaceous glands and is effective for both men and women.

Quercetin is a bioflavonoid that reduces inflammation

Probiotics: two capsules 3 times daily (especially, following the intake of antibiotics)

Milk Thistle detoxifies the liver, which may have been overstressed with toxins. Look for a product that is standardize 85 % silymarin content.

Dose: take 200 to 250 mg twice daily.

Neem detoxifies the liver, purifies the blood and a detoxicant. See my book on "Cholesterol."

Namely, **"Secretes To Lowering Cholesterol With Nutrition And Natural Supplements"**, Published by AuthorHouse.

Dandelion root (*Taraxacum officinale*) also supports liver detoxification. It is also a gentle laxative and can facilitate the elimination of waste. Use 300 to 500 mg in capsule form, 30 drops of tincture in water or 1 cup of tea three times daily.

Passionflower (*Passiflora incarnate*) and **Hops** (*Humulus lupulus*) is used when stress is causing your acne. Drink these calming teas whenever you need to wind down.

Chromium regulates blood sugar which can be beneficial for treating acne. Take 200 to 400 mcg daily.

Fibre Supplement: cleanses colon and eliminates constipation which are some of the contributing factors for acne and skin problems.

Dosage: 1 to 2 tsp psyllium husk fibre in 8 oz pure water. Drink plenty of water during the day.

Oil of Oregano kills yeast overgrowth associated with acne formation.

Colloidal silver has an antimicrobial property. Dab it onto pimples twice daily.

Natural progesterone cream is effective for pre menstrual and menopausal women

Herbs

Chamomile (*Matricaria recutita*): It is anti-inflammatory, and has soothing effects on the nervous system, as well.

Burdock root (*Arctium lappa*) Burdock root is used for purification and detoxification of blood. It has hormone balancing properties. It also improves elimination.

Dose: 300 to 500 mg, 30 drops of tincture, or 1 cup of tea three times daily.

Here is a Tea that may help purify the blood and Skin. Tea of Burdock root, Echinacea root, Dandelion root, Red Clover, yellow dock, and Sarsaparilla. Prepare by decoction using one ounce of this herb mix to three cups pure water. Simmer 20-25 minutes.

Dosage: Drink 8 oz three times daily between meals for a minimum of 10 weeks.

Goldenseal root (Hydrastis Canadensis) has detoxifying and antibacterial properties.

Dosage: 1 to 2 capsules or 30-50 drops extract in 4 ounce of water three times daily.

Gentian root (*Gentiana lutea*): Its beneficial property is: tonic bitter; traditionally used to aid digestion and elimination, and as a liver cleanser.

Dosage: Preferably use its extract, because actual perception of its bitter taste will in crease the body's response: 30-50 drops in 4 oz of pure water, three times daily.

Oregon Grape root (*Berberis aquifolium*): Its antibacterial properties may deter harmful bacterial growth in the large intestine and on the skin. It may also help as a blood purifier.

Dosage: 1 to 2 capsules or 30-50 drops extract in 4 oz water, three times daily.

Sunder Vati: An Ayurvedic formulation consisting of herbs Ginger, Holarrhena antidysenterica, and Embelia ribes has been shown to have significantly reduced both inflammatory and non-inflammatory lesions.

Herbal remedies such as aloe vera, horsetail, lemon balm, and tansy are commonly used for the treatment of acne. Some preparations made from these herbs may be used directly on the inflamed skin as topical treatments

Reduce Stress

Stress is the cause of various chronic diseases. It throws the body out of balance. Stress can affect skin by creating hormone imbalance, and disrupting digestion, elimination, and detoxification. Persons with acne are increasingly self-conscious about their looks. Techniques of stress reduction may ultimately help boost their self-esteem by improving skin health and appearance. Here are some of the relaxation techniques that can help to reduce stress.

- prayer, meditation, Kriya yoga, and pranayam
- exercise, massage therapy (Ayurvedic techniques are highly effective)
- **Hydrotherapy**: Epson Salt Bath (for people with heart conditions and diabetes are advised not to use Epson Salt Bath)

- **Acupressure**, acupuncture, and reflexology (consult professionals)
- **Biofeedback** and Guided imagery
- **Aromatherapy**: chose one or more of these essential oils. Geranium, Lavender, or Bergamot.

Bergamot; used for depression, stress, infection (all types of skin conditions, such acne, psoriasis, eczema). Its other therapeutic properties are: antiseptic, antibiotic, antispasmodic and antidepressant.

Geranium; used for depression, reduces inflammation, heals acne. It regulates the production of oil, and has rose-like aroma with minty undertones.

Lavender is calming to emotions and skin. It is used for acne, depression, itchy, scabies, scars, and sores.

Apply any one of these oils with a compress or put one or a combination of them in your bath. These oils are quite potent. You may try lightly one place first to find out its effect or dilute it with olive oil and apply. After the skin has improved, apply a lotion made with diluted water, lavender, and orange blossom to allay scaring.

Other Home Remedies Worth Looking At

Indian Acne Home Cure

Using water, make a paste with a teaspoon of turmeric powder and a teaspoon of sandalwood powder. Put it on acne and it will clear it up. This is a commonly used acne home remedy in India and you can get sandalwood powder online or from an Indian grocery.

Orange Peel Remedy

Finely grate an orange peel and mix it in water. Put this on your acne

Glycerin Soap Cure

Use glycerin soap. It will do away with the acne, the itchy skin, dryness and essentially you wind up with comfortable, beautiful skin. The glycerin soap alleviate itching and dryness on your skin. No more use of lotion on body or face to try to keep the skin moisturized. You don't have to put any oil on your face as it is perfectly balanced and your makeup looks good all day. Your skin will feel good instead of being painful and itchy.

Effective Home Remedies for Acne

Are you aware that your own toothpaste can be a major help in reducing the swelling of your pimples? Just apply it to the affected part before you sleep and in the morning you will see the instanteffect.

Chamomile Tea: A natural anti-inflammatory which will reduce acne flare-ups, it's antiseptic, antibacterial and antifungal. The chamomile tea bag should be soaked in lukewarm water and then apply to the skin for about 30 seconds. This will leave the skin and pores clean of excess oil and reduce skin inflammation and promote wound healing. As a drink Camomile tea is also associated with helping cure insomnia and easing headaches.

Sleep

your immune response to the infections that characterize Getting enough sleep is as vital for acne as it is for under-eye circles and wrinkles.

Especially for acne, lack of sufficient sleep may:

*Increase stress levels by making it much harder to cope with the stressors of daily life

*Trigger fluctuations in hormone levels that can lead to increased sebum production in many people

*reduce acne

Certainly, sleep needs vary according to the individual. Average optimal sleep ranges from 7.5-8.5 hours a night. Sleep is restorative as a time of growth and rejuvenation for the nervous and immune systems, and lack of sleep has been found to affect wound healing.

Also, what you sleep ON is important!

Change your pillowcase and bedding often, to substantially reduce bacteria. Oils and dead skin cells trapped in the fibers of bedding, creating a conducive environment for the growth of more bacteria, which then transfers back to your skin. If you really want to cut down on the bacteria where your face lies for a third of your day, use clean, white pillowcases that have been washed with bleach and rinsed well (so that residual bleach doesn't irritate your skin).

There are anti-bacterial pillows on the market which will take care of the bacteria issue under your pillowcase. Latex-made pillows are not only antibacterial and dust-roof, they have hundreds of holes in the foam that allow better air circulation throughout the night, don't allow moisture to build up, and provide support for a better night sleep.

Stern Advice:
-Never, ever touch your face.
- Use 3 facecloths to wash your face, one to soap on, one to soap off with very hot water, one to rinse off with ice cold water, in that order, once a day.
- If you are under 18 take 5,000 IU of vitamin A once a day with a full meal
- If you are over 18 take 5,000 IU of vitamin A twice a day with a full meal.
-Do not get pregnant while taking vitamin A. Do not take any more, like Accutane, it will stop you growing.
- Never, ever. pick, squeeze or pop your spot. Read the first above one again.

REFERENCE

1. Bassett, I. B. A comparative study of tea tree oil versus benzyl peroxide in the treatment of acne. Medical Journal of Australia. 1990; 153; 455-58.

2. Berkowsky, Bruce. Aromatherapy Synthesis Materia Medica. Mount Vernon, WA: Joseph Ben Hil-Meyer Research, 1999.

3. Boericke, William, M.D. Homeopathic Materia Medica National Homeo Laboratory, Calcutta.

4. Michaelsson, G., Vahlquist, A., Juhlin, L. Serum zinc and retinol binding protein in acne. Br J Dermatol. 1997; 96: 283-6.

5. Kugman, A., et al., Oral vitamin A in acne vulgaris. Int J Dermatol; 1981; 20: 278-85.

6. Questions and Answers About Acne. The National Institute of Arthritis and Musculoskeletal and Skin Diseases (NIAMS). National Institute of Health. Bethesda. January 2006. www.niams.nih.gov/hi/topics/acne/acne.htm

7. Paranjpe, P., Kulkarni, PH. Comparative efficacy of four Ayurvedic formulations in the treatment of acne vulgaris: a double-blind randomized placebo-controlled clinical evaluation. J Ethnopharm. 1995; 49: 127-132.

Check This Site Out for more info on Acne: http://amzn.to/y1nl02

Amazon Popular Products: http://bit.ly/z2qfMy

For Alternative Natural Remedies and Natural Cures Visit:

http://www.alternativenaturalremedies.com

To get into these sites use CTRL + enter

www.ingramcontent.com/pod-product-compliance
Lightning Source LLC
Chambersburg PA
CBHW070123010626
45794CB00012B/1246